# TABLE OF CONTENTS

1.INTRODUCTION 4
2.UNDERSTANDING WEIGHT LOSS 13
3.FOUNDATIONS OF A HEALTHY DIET 26
4. CREATING A BALANCED MEAL PLAN 35
5.ESSENTIAL NUTRIENTS FOR WEIGHT LOSS 46
6. MEAL PREPPING 56
7.OVERCOMING EMOTIONAL EATING AND OVERCOMING SETBACKS 66
8.MAXIMIZING WEIGHT LOSS WITH EXERCISE: TYPES AND BENEFITS 77
9.CUSTOMIZING NUTRITION AND MEAL PLANNING FOR INDIVIDUAL NEEDS 87
10.CONCLUSION 95

# INTRODUCTION

In a world where fad diets and quick-fix weight loss solutions dominate headlines and social media feeds, the importance of sustainable and scientifically sound nutrition practices cannot be overstated. Welcome to "Nutrition and Meal Planning for Weight Loss," a comprehensive guide that will empower you to take charge of your health, transform your eating habits, and achieve lasting weight loss results.

This book is designed to cut through the noise and provide you with the knowledge, strategies, and practical tools necessary to navigate the complex world of nutrition and meal planning. Whether you're starting your weight loss journey or looking to refine your current approach, this resource will be your trusted companion.

We understand that weight loss is a deeply personal and multifaceted endeavor, influenced by factors such as genetics, lifestyle, and individual circumstances. That's why this book takes a holistic approach, combining evidence-based nutrition principles with the art of meal planning to help you achieve sustainable results. We believe that nourishing your body and mind through balanced eating is not only the key to shedding excess weight but also the foundation for overall well-being.

Throughout these pages, we will debunk common myths, clarify misconceptions, and provide practical guidance rooted in scientific research. You will gain a deeper understanding of the fundamental components of a healthy diet, including macronutrients, portion control, and the power of mindful eating. Armed with this knowledge, you will be able to make informed choices about what and how much you eat, ensuring that your meals are both satisfying and supportive of your weight loss goals.

Creating a balanced meal plan is at the heart of successful weight loss. We will guide you through the process of setting realistic goals, determining your caloric needs, and designing meals that provide optimal nutrition while promoting fat loss. We will explore the vital role of essential nutrients, such as fiber, proteins, and healthy fats, and how they can enhance your weight loss journey.

Moreover, we understand that adopting a new way of eating can be challenging. That's why we will delve into the practical aspects of meal prepping and making smart food choices, equipping you with strategies to navigate social situations, dining out, and traveling while staying on track with your weight loss goals.

We also recognize that weight loss is not solely about the food we eat but also about our relationship with our bodies and the role of physical activity. We will explore how exercise complements proper nutrition, boost metabolism, and contributes to overall health and well-being.

Additionally, this book caters to various dietary preferences, dietary restrictions, and different age groups. We will provide guidance for individuals following vegetarian, vegan, or other specific dietary patterns, as well as those with medical conditions that require special attention.

Embarking on a weight loss journey is not always easy. Challenges may arise, setbacks may occur, and motivation may waver. But fear not! This book will offer guidance on overcoming obstacles, handling emotional eating, and maintaining long-term success. We believe in your ability to achieve your goals and create a healthier, happier version of yourself.

As you delve into the pages that follow, remember that this is not just a diet; it is a transformative journey towards a healthier lifestyle. We encourage you to embrace the information, implement the strategies, and customize your approach to suit your individual needs.

So, are you ready to revolutionize your relationship with food, unlock the power of nutrition, and embrace sustainable weight loss? Let's begin this exciting and rewarding journey together.

## 2.UNDERSTANDING WEIGHT LOSS

In a world where fad diets and quick-fix weight loss solutions dominate headlines and social media feeds, the importance of sustainable and scientifically sound nutrition practices cannot be overstated. Welcome to "Nutrition and

Meal Planning for Weight Loss," a comprehensive guide that will empower you to take charge of your health, transform your eating habits, and achieve lasting weight loss results.

This book is designed to cut through the noise and provide you with the knowledge, strategies, and practical tools necessary to navigate the complex world of nutrition and meal planning. Whether you're starting your weight loss journey or looking to refine your current approach, this resource will be your trusted companion.

We understand that weight loss is a deeply personal and multifaceted endeavor, influenced by factors such as genetics, lifestyle, and individual circumstances. That's why this book takes a holistic approach.

A. Explaining the Concept of Weight Loss:

Weight loss is a goal that many individuals strive to achieve, but it's essential to understand the underlying principles and mechanisms involved. In this chapter, we will delve into the concept of weight loss, exploring what it truly means and how it relates to your overall health.

Weight loss refers to the reduction of body weight, primarily through the loss of body fat. While it may seem simple on the surface—eat less, move more—there is much more to the process. Weight loss is a complex interplay of various factors, including nutrition, physical activity, metabolism, and individual differences.

We will explore the importance of setting realistic goals for weight loss, emphasizing the significance of sustainable and gradual progress. Rapid weight loss can be detrimental to your health and lead to muscle loss, nutrient deficiencies, and rebound weight gain. It's crucial to adopt a balanced and long-term approach to achieve lasting results.

## B. Factors Influencing Weight Loss:

Several key factors influence weight loss, and understanding them can help you navigate your journey more effectively. In this section, we will explore the factors that play a role in weight loss, including:

1. Calories: Calories are units of energy provided by the foods we consume. To lose weight, it's necessary to create a calorie deficit, which means consuming fewer calories than you expend. We will discuss the concept of energy balance and the importance of finding the right balance between calorie intake and expenditure.

2. Metabolism: Metabolism encompasses all the chemical processes in your body that convert food into energy. Your metabolic rate influences how

efficiently you burn calories. We will explore factors that affect metabolism, such as age, body composition, genetics, and lifestyle choices. Additionally, we will debunk common misconceptions about boosting metabolism and provide evidence-based strategies to support a healthy metabolism.

3. Nutrient Composition: While calorie balance is important, the quality of the calories you consume matters too. Different macronutrients

(carbohydrates, proteins, and fats) play unique roles in weight loss. We will discuss the impact of these macronutrients on satiety, energy levels, and overall health. Additionally, we will emphasize the significance of choosing nutrient-dense foods that provide essential vitamins, minerals, and fiber while keeping calorie intake in check.

C. Debunking Common Weight Loss Myths:

The weight loss industry is flooded with myths and misconceptions that can hinder progress and lead to frustration. In this section, we will debunk some of the most common weight loss myths, providing you with evidence-based information to separate fact from fiction. Some myths we will address include:

1. Myth: Crash diets are the most effective way to lose weight.
   - We will discuss the drawbacks of crash diets and

why they often lead to short-term results and long-term weight regain.

2. Myth: Eating fat makes you fat.
   - We will explore the importance of healthy fats in a balanced diet and how they can support weight loss efforts.

3. Myth: Carbohydrates should be completely eliminated.
   - We will address the role of carbohydrates, the importance of choosing the right types,

and debunk the idea that all carbs are "bad."

By dispelling these myths, you will be equipped with accurate information to make informed decisions about your nutrition and weight loss journey.

Understanding the concept of weight loss, recognizing the factors that influence it, and debunking common myths will provide a solid foundation for your journey towards a healthier weight. Armed with this knowledge, you will be better prepared to make sustainable choices and achieve your weight loss goals in a way that promotes overall well-being. In the following chapters, we will delve deeper into the practical aspects of creating a balanced meal plan and implementing effective strategies for weight loss success

# 3.FOUNDATIONS OF A HEALTHY DIET

As you embark on your weight loss journey, it's essential to establish a strong foundation for success. In this chapter, we will delve into the fundamental aspects of nutrition and meal planning, focusing on the role of macronutrients, the importance of portion control and mindful eating, and the incorporation of whole, nutrient-dense foods. By understanding and applying these principles, you will empower yourself to make informed choices, optimize your nutrition, and achieve your weight loss goals.

A. The Role of Macronutrients (Carbohydrates, Proteins, Fats)

Macronutrients, namely carbohydrates, proteins, and fats, are the building blocks of our diet. Each plays a unique role in our bodies and has specific implications for weight loss.

1. Carbohydrates:
Carbohydrates are a primary source of energy for our bodies. They can be classified into two categories: simple and complex. Simple carbohydrates, found in sugary drinks, sweets, and refined grains, are quickly digested, causing blood sugar spikes and crashes. Complex carbohydrates, found in whole grains, fruits, and vegetables,

provide a steady release of energy and are rich in fiber, vitamins, and minerals. When planning your meals, focus on incorporating complex carbohydrates while minimizing simple carbohydrates.

2. Proteins:

Proteins are the building blocks of our cells, tissues, and muscles. They play a crucial role in repairing and maintaining our bodies. Protein-rich foods such as lean meats, fish, poultry, legumes, and dairy products promote satiety, increase metabolism, and preserve lean muscle mass during weight loss. Aim to include a moderate serving of protein in each meal to support your weight loss journey effectively.

3. Fats:

Fats are often misunderstood and unfairly demonized. While it's true that fats are high in calories, they are essential for various bodily functions and overall well-being. Healthy fats, such as those found in avocados, nuts, seeds, and olive oil, provide essential fatty acids and fat-soluble vitamins. They also aid in satiety, making you feel fuller for longer periods. When incorporating fats into your meal plan, focus on consuming unsaturated fats while limiting saturated and trans fats.

B. Importance of Portion Control and Mindful Eating

In our fast-paced society, we often consume meals

mindlessly, unaware of portion sizes or the cues our bodies give us. Portion control and mindful eating can transform the way we interact with food, leading to improved weight loss outcomes and overall well-being.

1. Portion Control:
Portion control involves being mindful of the amount of food you eat at each meal or snack. It helps prevent overeating and allows you to enjoy a wide variety of foods without exceeding your calorie needs.

Use visual cues, such as measuring cups, to understand appropriate portion sizes. Additionally, listen to your body's hunger and fullness signals, stopping when you feel comfortably satisfied.

## 2. Mindful Eating:

Mindful eating encourages a non-judgmental awareness of the present moment's food experience. It involves paying attention to the taste, texture, and aroma of each bite, as well as your body's hunger and satiety cues. By slowing down and savoring your meals, you can develop a healthier relationship with food, reduce emotional eating, and make conscious choices that support your weight loss goals.

## C. Incorporating Whole, Nutrient-Dense Foods

When it comes to weight loss, not all foods are created equal. Prioritizing whole, nutrient-dense foods is crucial for achieving optimal health and sustainable weight loss.

## 1. Whole Foods:

Whole foods are minimally processed and retain their natural nutrient content

# 4. CREATING A BALANCED MEAL PLAN

## Section A: Setting Realistic Goals

When setting weight loss goals, it is essential to be practical and consider various factors. Here are some guidelines to help you set realistic goals:

1. Assess Your Starting Point: Take an honest look at your current weight, body composition, and overall health. Consult with a healthcare professional to determine a healthy weight range for your body type and height.

2. Gradual Approach: Aim for a gradual and sustainable weight loss of 1-2 pounds per week. Rapid weight loss can often lead to muscle loss and a higher likelihood of regaining the weight.

3. Behavior-based Goals: Instead of solely focusing on the number on the scale, consider setting behavior-based goals. Examples include eating five servings of vegetables daily, exercising for at least 30 minutes five times a

week, or reducing your intake of sugary beverages.

4. Non-Scale Victories: Celebrate non-scale victories such as increased energy levels, improved sleep quality, or enhanced self-confidence. These achievements can be powerful motivators on your weight loss journey.

Section B: Determining Caloric Needs for Weight Loss Understanding your caloric needs is essential when it comes to effective weight loss.

Here's how you can determine the appropriate calorie intake:

1. Basal Metabolic Rate (BMR): Calculate your BMR, which represents the number of calories your body needs to maintain basic bodily functions at rest. There are several online calculators available to estimate your BMR based on factors like age, gender, height, and weight.

2. Caloric Deficit: To lose weight, create a caloric deficit by consuming fewer calories

than your body needs. Start with a modest deficit of 500-750 calories per day, as extreme deficits can be unsustainable and may lead to nutrient deficiencies.

3. Individual Variations: Keep in mind that everyone's metabolism is unique, and these calculations provide a general guideline. Adjustments may be necessary based on factors like activity level, muscle mass, and specific health conditions.

## Section C: Designing a Balanced Plate: Proportions and Food Groups

Achieving a balanced plate is crucial for providing your body with the necessary nutrients while promoting weight loss. Consider the following tips:

1. Portion Control: Practice portion control by dividing your plate into specific proportions. Fill half of your plate with non-starchy vegetables, one-quarter with lean protein sources, and the remaining

quarter with whole grains or starchy vegetables.

2. Include Healthy Fats: Don't shy away from incorporating healthy fats, such as avocados, nuts, and olive oil, into your meals. They provide satiety and essential nutrients.

3. Focus on Fiber: Include high-fiber foods like fruits, vegetables, whole grains, and legumes. Fiber helps you feel fuller for longer, aids in digestion, and promotes overall well-being.

4. Hydration: Remember to stay hydrated by drinking water throughout the day. Sometimes, thirst can be mistaken for hunger, leading to unnecessary calorie consumption.

Section D: Meal Planning Strategies and Tips
Meal planning is a valuable tool for weight loss success. Consider the following strategies and tips to make the most of your meal planning efforts:

1. Plan Ahead: Dedicate some time each week to plan your meals and snacks. This helps you make healthier choices and reduces

 the likelihood of impulsive, less nutritious options.

2. Variety and Balance: Aim for a variety of foods from different food groups to ensure you obtain a broad range of nutrients. Experiment with new recipes, flavors, and cooking

methods to keep your meals exciting.

3. Preparing in Advance: Consider prepping ingredients or even whole meals in advance. Having healthy, portion-controlled options readily available can help you avoid unhealthy temptations.

4. Mindful Eating: Practice mindful eating by savoring each bite, paying attention to your body's hunger and fullness cues, and eating without distractions. This

approach encourages a healthier relationship with food and prevents overeating.

## 5.ESSENTIAL NUTRIENTS FOR WEIGHT LOSS

In your journey towards weight loss, optimizing your nutrition is key to achieving sustainable and long-term success. In this chapter, we will explore the importance of fiber in promoting satiety and digestion, the significance of lean proteins for muscle preservation and metabolism, the role of healthy fats in hormone regulation and satiety, and the impact of micronutrients on overall health and weight management. By understanding and incorporating these elements into your meal planning, you can elevate your nutrition and enhance your weight loss efforts.

## A. Importance of Fiber in Promoting Satiety and Digestion

1. Satiety: High-fiber foods have the remarkable ability to keep you feeling full and satisfied for longer periods. Fiber adds bulk to your meals, slows down digestion, and promotes a sense of satiety. Incorporating fiber-rich foods like fruits, vegetables, whole grains, legumes, and nuts into your meals can help you manage hunger and reduce overall calorie intake.

2. Digestion: Fiber plays a crucial role in maintaining a healthy digestive system. It adds bulk to stools, promotes regular bowel movements, and prevents constipation. Aim to include a variety of soluble and insoluble fiber sources in your diet to support optimal digestive function.

B. The Significance of Lean Proteins for Muscle Preservation and Metabolism

1. Muscle Preservation: During weight loss, it is essential to preserve muscle mass as it contributes to overall metabolic rate. Lean proteins, such as skinless poultry, fish, lean meats, tofu, and legumes, provide the necessary amino acids to support muscle preservation. Including adequate protein in your meals can also help you feel fuller and satisfied, preventing overeating.

2. Metabolism: Protein has a higher thermic effect

compared to carbohydrates and fats, meaning it requires more energy to digest and metabolize. By incorporating lean proteins into your meal plan, you can slightly increase your metabolic rate and support your weight loss efforts.

## C. Healthy Fats and Their Role in Hormone Regulation and Satiety

1. Hormone Regulation: Healthy fats, such as those found in avocados, nuts,

seeds, and olive oil, play a vital role in hormone regulation. They provide essential fatty acids that help produce and balance hormones necessary for metabolism, satiety, and overall well-being. Including moderate amounts of healthy fats in your meals can support hormonal balance and optimize weight management.

2. Satiety: Fats contribute to the feeling of satiety and help you stay satisfied between meals. Including a small

serving of healthy fats in your meals, such as a tablespoon of nut butter or a drizzle of olive oil, can enhance the flavor of your dishes and promote a sense of fullness.

D. Micronutrients and Their Impact on Overall Health and Weight Management

1. Overall Health: Micronutrients, including vitamins and minerals, are essential for overall health and well-being. They play a vital role in supporting various

bodily functions, including metabolism, energy production, immune system function, and cell regeneration. A balanced diet rich in fruits, vegetables, whole grains, lean proteins, and healthy fats can provide a wide array of micronutrients necessary for optimal health.

2. Weight Management: Micronutrient deficiencies can impact weight management. Certain micronutrients, such as vitamin D, iron, and B vitamins, are involved in

energy metabolism and can affect your body's ability to efficiently use and burn calories. Ensure you consume a diverse range of nutrient-dense foods to meet your micronutrient needs and support healthy weight management.

By focusing on the importance of fiber, lean proteins, healthy fats, and micronutrients in your nutrition.

# 6. MEAL PREPPING

Meal prepping and making healthier choices while dining out or traveling are essential components of a successful weight loss journey. In this chapter, we will explore the benefits of meal prepping, strategies for planning and preparing meals in advance, and tips for making healthier food choices when dining out or traveling. By implementing these strategies, you can simplify your nutrition and stay on track with your weight loss goals, even in busy and challenging situations.

## A. Benefits of Meal Prepping for Weight Loss

1. Portion Control: Meal prepping allows you to portion your meals in advance, ensuring that you consume the appropriate amount of calories and nutrients. By controlling portion sizes, you can avoid overeating and maintain a calorie deficit for weight loss.

2. Time and Convenience: Meal prepping saves time and effort throughout the week. By dedicating a few hours to preparing meals in advance, you eliminate the need for daily cooking and decision-making. This convenience reduces the chances of opting for unhealthy, fast-food options when you're short on time.

3. Nutritional Balance: When you plan and prepare your meals, you have control over the ingredients and their

nutritional content. You can create balanced meal that include lean proteins, whole grains, healthy fats, and a variety of fruits and vegetables. This balanced approach ensures that you meet your nutrient needs while promoting weight loss.

## B. Planning and Preparing Meals in Advance

1. Meal Planning: Start by creating a meal plan for the week. Consider your caloric needs, macronutrient

requirements, and personal preferences. Plan meals that can be easily batch cooked or assembled ahead of time.

2. Batch Cooking: Choose a day or two each week to dedicate to cooking and preparing meals in bulk. Cook proteins, grains, and roasted vegetables that can be portioned and stored for later use. This way, you'll have ready-to-eat components to assemble balanced meals throughout the week.

3. Portioning and Storage: After cooking, portion your meals into individual containers or reusable bags. Label them with the contents and date to keep track of freshness. Store them in the refrigerator or freezer based on your consumption timeline.

C. Strategies for Healthier Food Choices when Dining Out or Traveling

1. Plan Ahead: Before dining out or traveling, research the available restaurant options or

check the menu online. Look for healthier choices that align with your weight loss goals, such as grilled proteins, steamed vegetables, or salads. Having a plan in place helps you make informed decisions and avoid impulsive choices.

2. Mindful Eating: Practice mindful eating when dining out or traveling. Pay attention to your hunger and fullness cues, eat slowly, and savor each bite. Avoid distractions like electronic devices and focus

on enjoying the food and the company.

3. Modifications and Substitutions: Don't hesitate to make requests for modifications or substitutions to make your meals healthier. Ask for dressings or sauces on the side, opt for grilled or baked options instead of fried, and choose whole grain alternatives when available.

4. Smart Snacking: When traveling, pack nutritious snacks like fruits, nuts, or

protein bars to avoid relying on unhealthy options available on the go. Having healthy snacks on hand can help you resist temptations and stay on track with your weight loss goals.

By incorporating meal prepping into your routine and adopting strategies for healthier choices while dining out or traveling, you can maintain consistency and support your weight loss efforts even in challenging situations. These practices will simplify your nutrition and empower you to make informed decisions that align with your goals.


NUTRITION AND MEAL PLANNING FOR WEIGHT LOSS     1

A Detailed Step Step Book on How To Lose Weight Effectively     1

By     1

**INTRODUCTION**     **4**

**2.UNDERSTANDING WEIGHT LOSS**     **12**

**3.FOUNDATIONS OF A HEALTHY DIET**     **25**

**4. CREATING A BALANCED MEAL PLAN**     **34**

**5.ESSENTIAL NUTRIENTS FOR WEIGHT LOSS**     **45**

**6. MEAL PREPPING**     **55**

**7.OVERCOMING EMOTIONAL EATING AND OVERCOMING SETBACKS**     **65**

**8.MAXIMIZING WEIGHT LOSS WITH EXERCISE:**

TYPES AND BENEFITS     76
9.CUSTOMIZING NUTRITION AND MEAL PLANNING FOR INDIVIDUAL NEEDS     86
10.CONCLUSION     94


# 7.OVERCOMING EMOTIONAL EATING AND OVERCOMING SETBACKS

In the pursuit of weight loss, it's crucial to address emotional eating, maintain motivation, and navigate through setbacks and plateaus. This chapter will explore effective strategies for overcoming emotional eating and cravings, staying motivated for long-term success, and handling setbacks and plateaus. By equipping yourself with the right tools, you can overcome challenges and continue progressing on your weight loss journey.

A. Dealing with Emotional Eating and Cravings

1. Recognize Triggers: Identify the triggers that lead to emotional eating, such as stress, boredom, or certain

situations. Awareness is the first step in breaking the cycle. Keep a journal to track your emotions and the circumstances surrounding your cravings.

2. Find Alternative Coping Mechanisms: Instead of turning to food, explore alternative coping mechanisms to address emotions. Engage in activities that bring you joy or help you relax, such as reading, practicing mindfulness, going for a walk,

or talking to a supportive friend or family member.

3. Mindful Eating: Practice mindful eating to build a healthier relationship with food. Slow down, savor each bite, and pay attention to hunger and fullness cues. By eating with intention and awareness, you can distinguish between physical hunger and emotional cravings.

4. Seek Support: Consider seeking support from a

therapist, counselor, or support group specializing in emotional eating. They can provide guidance, tools, and a safe space to explore and overcome emotional triggers.

B. Strategies for Staying Motivated and Maintaining Long-Term Success

1. Set Realistic and Meaningful Goals: Set goals that are achievable, measurable, and personally meaningful. Break them down into smaller milestones to track

your progress and celebrate achievements along the way.

2. Find Intrinsic Motivation: Identify your intrinsic motivations for losing weight, such as improved health, increased energy, or enhanced self-confidence. Connect with these motivations regularly to stay focused and committed.

3. Celebrate Non-Scale Victories: Shift your focus from solely relying on the scale. Celebrate non-scale victories,

such as fitting into smaller clothes, improved strength, increased stamina, or positive changes in mood and overall well-being.

4. Accountability and Support: Find an accountability partner or join a weight loss support group. Sharing your goals, challenges, and successes with others can provide encouragement, advice, and a sense of community.

C. Handling Setbacks and Plateaus in Weight Loss

1. Reframe Setbacks: Instead of viewing setbacks as failures, reframe them as learning opportunities. Understand that setbacks are a normal part of the journey and can provide valuable insights and lessons for future success.

2. Assess and Adjust: When faced with a plateau or setback, evaluate your current approach. Are there any areas where you can make adjustments? Assess your

nutrition, exercise routine, stress levels, and sleep quality. Make necessary changes to jumpstart progress.

3. Focus on Non-Scale Progress: During plateaus, shift your focus to non-scale progress. Look for improvements in body composition, energy levels, fitness performance, or overall well-being. Celebrate these victories and remember that weight loss is not the only indicator of success.

4.     Seek     Professional Guidance:      If      you're experiencing          prolonged plateaus   or   struggling   to navigate   setbacks,   consider consulting     a     registered dietitian     or     healthcare professional   specializing   in weight management. They can provide          personalized guidance,  tailored  strategies, and   help   you   overcome obstacles.

Remember,  weight  loss  is  a journey  with  ups  and  downs. By     addressing     emotional eating, staying motivated, and handling setbacks and plateaus, you can build resilience, maintain progress, and achieve long-term success on your path to a healthier lifestyle.

# 8.MAXIMIZING WEIGHT LOSS WITH EXERCISE: TYPES AND BENEFITS

In your quest for optimal weight loss, incorporating exercise alongside a healthy nutrition plan is essential. In this chapter, we will explore the importance of complementing nutrition with exercise for weight loss and delve into the various types of exercise and their impact on metabolism and body composition. By understanding the benefits of different exercise modalities, you can create a well-rounded fitness routine that enhances your weight loss efforts.

A. Complementing Nutrition with Exercise for Optimal Weight Loss

1. Caloric Expenditure: Exercise increases energy expenditure, allowing you to create a greater calorie deficit. When combined with a well-balanced nutrition plan,

exercise can accelerate weight loss by burning additional calories.

2. Muscle Preservation: Regular exercise, particularly resistance training, helps preserve and build lean muscle mass. Muscle is metabolically active, meaning it burns more calories at rest than fat. By incorporating exercise, you can support muscle preservation and prevent muscle loss during weight loss.

3. Health Benefits: Exercise offers numerous health benefits, including improved cardiovascular health, enhanced mood, increased energy levels, and reduced risk of chronic diseases. These benefits contribute to an overall sense of well-being and support long-term weight management.

B. Types of Exercise and Their Impact on Metabolism and Body Composition

1.       Aerobic/Cardiovascular Exercise: Aerobic exercises, such as running, cycling, swimming, or brisk walking, increase heart rate and oxygen consumption. These activities primarily enhance cardiovascular health, burn calories, and improve endurance. While aerobic exercise alone may not significantly alter body composition, it plays a valuable role in calorie expenditure and overall health.

2.     Resistance     Training: Resistance training, including weightlifting, bodyweight exercises, or resistance bands, stimulates muscle growth and strength development. It helps increase muscle mass, which can elevate your resting metabolic rate and promote fat loss. Resistance training also improves body composition by shaping and toning your physique.

3.     High-Intensity     Interval Training (HIIT): HIIT involves

alternating periods of high-intensity exercise with short recovery periods. It boosts cardiovascular fitness, burns calories, and can be an efficient way to increase metabolism and promote fat loss. HIIT workouts are typically shorter in duration but provide a significant afterburn effect, where your body continues burning calories post-exercise.

4. Flexibility and Balance Exercises: While flexibility and balance exercises, such as

yoga or Pilates, may not have a direct impact on weight loss, they contribute to overall fitness and well-being. These exercises improve mobility, posture, and body awareness, which can enhance your overall fitness journey and reduce the risk of injuries.

5. Incorporating Variety: Incorporating a mix of different exercise modalities is beneficial for weight loss and overall fitness. It prevents boredom, challenges your body in different ways, and

maximizes the benefits of both aerobic and resistance training. Consider combining different exercises throughout the week to keep your routine exciting and effective.

Remember to consult with a healthcare professional before starting a new exercise program, especially if you have any underlying health conditions or injuries. Gradually increase the intensity and duration of your workouts to avoid overexertion.

By complementing your nutrition plan with exercise, you can enhance weight loss, promote muscle preservation, and improve overall health. Understanding the impact of different exercise types on metabolism and body composition allows you to tailor your fitness routine to meet your specific goals. Embrace the joy of movement, find activities you enjoy, and make exercise an integral part of your weight loss journey.

# 9.CUSTOMIZING NUTRITION AND MEAL PLANNING FOR INDIVIDUAL NEEDS

In this chapter, we will explore the importance of customizing nutrition and meal planning to accommodate specific dietary preferences, dietary restrictions or medical conditions, as well as different age groups. By tailoring your approach to these individual needs, you can optimize weight loss efforts while ensuring optimal health and satisfaction.

## A. Nutrition and Meal Planning for Specific Dietary Preferences

1. Vegetarian and Vegan Diets: For individuals following a vegetarian or vegan diet, it's important to ensure adequate intake of essential nutrients such as protein, iron, calcium, and vitamin B12. Incorporate plant-based protein sources

like legumes, tofu, tempeh, and quinoa. Include a variety of fruits, vegetables, whole grains, and fortified plant-based alternatives to meet nutritional needs.

2.	Gluten-Free	Diets: Individuals with gluten sensitivity or celiac disease should avoid gluten-containing grains such as wheat, barley, and rye. Focus on naturally gluten-free whole grains like rice, quinoa, oats (certified gluten-free), and corn. Ensure proper label reading to avoid hidden sources of gluten in processed foods.

B. Meal Planning for Individuals with Dietary Restrictions or Medical Conditions

1. Diabetes: Individuals with diabetes benefit from meal planning that promotes stable blood sugar levels. Emphasize a balanced plate with controlled portions of carbohydrates, lean proteins, and healthy fats. Incorporate high-fiber foods, such as

whole grains, legumes, and non-starchy vegetables, and limit added sugars and refined carbohydrates.

2. Food Allergies and Intolerances: For individuals with food allergies or intolerances, careful attention must be given to ingredient selection and cross-contamination prevention. Substitute allergenic ingredients with suitable alternatives and consider working with a registered dietitian to ensure a

nutritionally balanced and safe meal plan.

## C. Tailoring Nutrition and Meal Planning for Different Age Groups

1. Children and Adolescents: Proper nutrition is crucial for growth and development in children and adolescents. Focus on nutrient-dense foods, including whole grains, lean proteins, fruits, vegetables, and dairy (or dairy alternatives). Encourage regular meals and snacks to

support energy needs and limit intake of processed foods and sugary beverages.

2. Older Adults: As individuals age, nutrient needs may change. Encourage a varied diet with a focus on lean proteins, high-fiber foods, and sources of calcium and vitamin D for bone health. Adequate hydration and portion control are important considerations. Working with a healthcare professional or registered dietitian can help address

specific needs and ensure optimal nutrition.

When tailoring nutrition and meal planning to individual needs, it's crucial to consider nutrient requirements, personal preferences, and any potential health concerns. Consulting with a registered dietitian or healthcare professional can provide personalized guidance and support.

By customizing meal plans to specific dietary preferences,

restrictions, and age groups, you can ensure that your weight loss journey aligns with your individual needs, promoting long-term success and optimal health. Remember, a sustainable approach is key, and finding enjoyment in the foods you consume plays a significant role in maintaining healthy habits for life.

## 10.CONCLUSION

Congratulations! You have reached the end of this book

on nutrition and meal planning for weight loss. Throughout this journey, we have explored the fundamental principles of nutrition, the role of macronutrients, portion control, incorporating whole foods, meal prepping, and so much more. Now, it's time to recap the key takeaways, provide encouragement for your weight loss journey, and offer resources for further information and support.

A. Recap of Key Takeaways

1. Balanced Nutrition: Focus on a well-balanced diet that includes all macronutrients (carbohydrates, proteins, and fats) and incorporates nutrient-dense whole foods.

2. Portion Control: Practice portion control to manage calorie intake and create a calorie deficit for weight loss. Use tools like measuring cups, food scales, or visual references to guide your portion sizes.

3. Mindful Eating: Develop mindful eating habits to foster a healthy relationship with food. Pay attention to hunger and fullness cues, savor each bite, and be aware of emotional triggers that may lead to overeating.

4. Meal Prepping: Embrace the benefits of meal prepping, such as saving time, promoting healthier choices, and ensuring consistency in your nutrition plan. Plan and prepare your meals in advance

to support your weight loss goals.

5. Making Healthy Choices: Opt for nutrient-dense foods, such as fruits, vegetables, whole grains, lean proteins, and healthy fats. Be mindful of added sugars, processed foods, and unhealthy fats.

6. Exercise and Movement: Combine your nutrition plan with regular physical activity to enhance weight loss, preserve muscle mass, boost

metabolism, and improve overall health.

## B. Encouragement for Your Weight Loss Journey

Embarking on a weight loss journey can be challenging, but it is also a transformative and empowering experience. Remember that your goals are within reach, and every small step forward counts. Stay motivated, stay consistent, and believe in your ability to create positive change.

Celebrate each milestone along the way, whether it's shedding a few pounds, fitting into smaller clothes, or feeling more energized and confident. Your commitment to your health and well-being is worth it, and the benefits will extend far beyond just weight loss.

C. Resources and References for Further Information and Support

As you continue your weight loss journey, it's important to have access to reliable resources and support. Here are some references and tools that can provide further information and assistance:

1. Books: Explore reputable books on nutrition, weight loss, and meal planning to deepen your knowledge. Look for evidence-based information and recommendations from trusted authors and experts.

2. Websites and Online Resources: Utilize reputable websites and online platforms that offer guidance on

nutrition, meal planning, exercise routines, and healthy recipes. Look for sources backed by registered dietitians, nutritionists, and healthcare professionals.

3. Registered Dietitians and Nutritionists: Consider seeking personalized guidance from a registered dietitian or nutritionist. They can provide tailored meal plans, address specific dietary concerns, and offer ongoing support throughout your weight loss journey.

4.     Support     Groups     and Communities:  Join  local  or online  support  groups  where you     can     connect     with individuals  who  are  also  on  a weight  loss  journey.  Sharing experiences,  challenges,  and successes        can        provide encouragement              and motivation.

Remember,  this  book  is  just the  beginning  of  your  lifelong commitment  to  healthy  eating and  weight  management.  Be open  to  learning,  adapt  as needed, and find what works best for you. With dedication, patience, and the right tools, you have the power to achieve your weight loss goals and embrace a healthier, happier life.

Wishing you success and fulfillment on your weight loss journey!